HOW TO LOOSE WEIGHT NATURALLY

A FRUIT AND VEGETABLE DIET

TABLE OF CONTENT

INTRODUCTION

Ask with respect to whether they need to get fit as a fiddle and you will see 100 hands go up. Ask those comparable hundred people how to get more slender and you will see a restriction of five hands. The reality of the situation is, various people need to get fit as a fiddle, yet not very many ability to do it.

So what's the issue with getting fit as a fiddle? There are various reasons why people may have to decrease their weight. Some may require it for prosperity reasons. As a matter of fact strength can provoke huge clinical issues like diabetes, coronary disease, and stroke, so those at high risk for developing any of these infections should consider a weight decrease schedule. Others need to get fit as a fiddle basically in light of the fact that they could do without the way where they look. While there is nothing out of order with several pounds, many take the prospect of weight decrease to unsafe furthest reaches that consolidate dangerous eating regimens and exercise routines Diet: Dieting despite a standard exercise routine will help you shed unwanted pounds. There are many eating routine undertakings out there, so it's connected to picking one that works. The best way to deal with finish up is to guide a subject matter expert or even someone you understand who has been on a tight eating schedule. You will really need to find what the eating routine surmises and if it is sensible for you.

CHAPTER ONE
A PLANT BASED FOOD

When was the last time you attempted another eating regimen and felt extraordinary, had the opportunity to eat what you adored, and effectively shed pounds? It might have never occurred. Most weight control plans leave you feeling eager, denied and afterward when you unavoidably "cheat" and eat fulfilling food, you end up crushed.

However it is conceivable to top off on sound, fulfilling nourishments, have energy, and effectively get thinner, as p

er sustenance master a Registered Dietician who made The VegStart Diet as a method of assisting you with getting in shape the solid way, while as yet eating what you love, and topping off on plant-based suppers and tidbits that are so loaded with solid fixings, empowering cell reinforcements and filling fiber, that you never feel denied, eager or languid, and you shed pounds in a feasible way that makes it simple to keep it off.

A notable nutritionist, made solid, filling, low-calorie plans for the VegStart Diet, which are intended to assist you with shedding pounds while eating the nourishments you love, similar to pasta and bread, comfort food like soup, and even delectable sweet or crunchy snacks. The plans are scrumptious. outrageous eating fewer carbs isn't neccessary, considers the VegStart a "practical health improvement plan," so there's no concern of going hungry.

Beside the eating regimen questions, specialist said reality with regards to the significance of extravagances like wine, chocolate, and treats. they shared their go-to swindle suppers, how to treat yourself the solid way, in addition to the most delectable plant-based proteins, and the most valuable fixings that everybody ought to have available. On the off chance that this is your first way to deal with a plant-based eating routine or you began eating plant-based some time back, when meat choices weren't anywhere near, you most likely have a great deal of inquiries.

What is The VegStart Diet? Is it a detox? Is it a program anybody can do whenever?

I don't have confidence in limits. I put stock in feasible changes. I have a great deal of discussions with individuals today about this theme. In case we're hoping to get in shape, The VegStart diet program is intended for weight reduction yet unquestionably, everybody's individual necessities are unique. The eating regimen centers around supportable weight reduction that is as yet going to keep you feeling fulfilled and meet your sustenance needs since we would prefer not to become supplement lacking when we're kind of attempting to follow something. There's very a way of life change angle to the eating routine in case you're not plant-based as of now.

What are the medical advantages of going plant-based.

It's an incredible proof based method of eating that has been appeared to lessen the danger of different conditions like cardiovascular diseases, and number of tumors. I'm working low maintenance at the clinic in the malignant growth care centers. Along these lines, I manage individuals regularly who have different judgments and I suggest those patients eat plant-based nourishments.

It very well may be overpowering to discover various approaches to cook those plant-based proteins and how to consolidate them into your family's suppers, yet discover those proteins you like and spotlight on fusing them into your eating regimen.

Presumably my most loved is tempeh, trailed by tofu which is a major one, and edamame...I love the simplicity of cooking it like commonly I get it frozen. I may very well defrost it or put it in like a sautéed food.

TOP FIVE FLAVORS THAT YOU GENERALLY HAVE AVALIABLE.

I'd need to say basil and oregano. Those are unquestionably my go-to flavors. I additionally love paprika, cumin, and cinnamon. I positively have a sweet tooth so I like to add cinnamon into my overnight oats. I like the smoky kinds of cumin and paprika on my tempeh.

there is a particular enhancement you take that is deficient in a plant-based eating routine

A B12 supplement and an iron enhancement. That is to say, since you follow a plant-based doesn't mean you will be low in iron. Along these lines, its kind of at a higher danger for iron insufficiency.

Yet, you can likewise get the B12 from dietary yeast and plant-based milk as opposed to taking an enhancement. At times I will take a plant-based omega-3 enhancement, however once more, you can get omega-3s in flaxseeds, chia seeds, and pecans. The reality is, you positively don't need to enhance, you can get enough supplements through food—yet those are only ones I take for additional confirmation.

Would it be a good idea for us to dodge treats?

At whatever point we're getting a charge out of sweets, I call them fun suppers. They sure don't have a huge load of supplements as our different dinners do, yet at whatever point we're appreciating them, eat them without blame since, supposing that we have blame we will not have

11

acknowledgment at that point that is the point at which it transforms into you eating the entire sack of chips or chocolates. At the point when we have a positive outlook on eating something we're probably going to recognize it snappier. I typically say to focus on 90% customary dinners and 10% fun suppers. It's alright to have a great time dinners each week, and the rest ought to be solid suppers. Certainly leave some space for un!

Tips for weight reduction

The greatest thing you need to do is to feel satiated. Obviously, you need to meet those supplement needs since we're not going to hit those drawn out weight reduction objectives in case we're feeling denied. Whatever changes you will make, simply ensure you can support them. I see such countless individuals in my training that are yo-yo weight watchers surrender. That cycle will proceed in the event that we do things that are along these lines, so prohibitive. I saw somebody yesterday in my training who was eating one feast a day, just, that is it. That framework worked for them, however, for a great many people, that won't be reasonable.

Going plant-based isn't costly

Not really. In case you're eating an entire food plant-based eating routine, you're eating beans and tofu for protein, and tofu costs $1 or $2 for a square, and you can get beans for not exactly a dollar. In the event that you live in a hotter environment you clearly have better admittance to new deliver lasting through the year, however it's alright if to utilize frozen produce as I do on the grounds that I live in Canada. I believe it's less expensive to eat plant-based and it's an incredible method to set aside cash. Proceed with the diet,the most amazing aspect is, you can continue to blend those plans into your everyday daily schedule and utilize those exercises and tips you gained from The VegStart diet. On the off chance that you began feast preparing and arranging, continue to go with that. The calorie level of the eating regimen is around 1,400 every day and if that works for you, keep doing that get you can generally make alterations to the plans. I would suggest making more plant-based suppers. The Beet posts new plans each day so you know where you can get them. Attempt to make a plant-based eating regimen part of your way of life.

By and by, when I previously went plant-based, around 10 years prior or something like that, I had a sluggish progress yet it just required a month in the wake of eating this approach to feel a recognizable distinction.

CHAPTER TWO
PAPAYA

Add Papaya to Your Smoothie to reduce Disease and Fight Aging

In the event that you imagine that papaya is just a warm-climate natural product, or to be delighted in an extended get-away in a tropical heaven with a cut of mint, you're passing up the astonishing advantages the splendid orange organic product has to bring to the table. Studies show that papaya, with its lycopene-filled tissue, pack`s in a greater number of cancer prevention agents and nutrients per 100 grams than practically some other organic product. Lycopene is known to diminish aggravation connected to significant sicknesses, and eating a high-lycopene diet helps bring down your danger of specific diseases and shields your skin from sun harm and early indications of maturing.

Studies likewise propose that eating lycopene helps battle irritation, which adds to ongoing illnesses like coronary illness, type 2 diabetes, joint inflammation, Crohn's infection, and then some. In any case, that is not by any means the only motivation to cherish papaya.

Pregnant Women Should Avoid Papaya Seeds and Unripe Papaya

Unripe or green papaya contains undeniable levels of what's called papaya latex, a smooth fluid that can be conceivably unsafe to pregnant ladies since it has been known to prompt uterine constrictions. The seeds are likewise known to spike withdrawals so on the off chance that you are pregnant, specialists caution you to not eat papaya.

Papaya is a top pick for any individual who loves tropical organic product since it's a blend among melon and mango, with a milder surface, and a spread like consistency that softens in your mouth. On the off chance that you discover it excessively rich, blend it into smoothies and use it to improve any formula rather than other juice.

Here are the 5 science-supported medical advantages of papaya

1. Papaya is Highly Nutritious and Low in Calories

A big part of little papaya contains more nutrient c than a solitary orange. It has 87 milligrams for every cup or 157% of your suggested day by day prerequisite of nutrient C, so eating papaya in the virus cold weather months is a safe sponsor.

A big part of little papaya likewise contains 33% of your suggested every day necessity of Vitamin A, which is additionally extraordinary for invulnerability, just as visual perception. A similar half papaya will convey 14% of your suggested necessity of Vitamin B9, which helps uphold sound cell work. This folate nutrient additionally will help you feel less slow.

Papaya completes this effectively, with just 62 calories in a cup, which is incredibly low for sweet organic product. Papaya is a decent wellspring of fiber, pressing in almost 3 grams for each serving. Since most natural products don't contain protein, papaya is extraordinary in that it contains 1 gram of plant-based protein.

2. Papaya Contains Lycopene, a Powerful Antioxidant That Lowers Cancer Risk

Studies show that the lycopene in papaya shields your body from harm brought about by free extremists. Consider free extremists negative particles that cause inconvenience, and the cell reinforcements as sure powers that kill them. By eating lycopene you bring down your degrees of oxidative pressure, which is connected to constant infections, like a few malignant growths, type 2 diabetes, coronary illness, and Alzheimer's, as per this investigation. By eating food sources containing lycopene like tomatoes, watermelon, guava, and papaya, you shield your body from the danger of infection.

Another investigation showed that "higher lycopene utilization was straightly connected with a diminished danger of prostate disease," and the examination additionally expressed: "there was a pattern that with higher lycopene admission, there were decreased occurrence of prostate malignant growth."

3. Papaya Helps Fight Inflammation that Causes Disease. 2 Servings a Day is Enough

Constant aggravation is a main source of numerous way of life sicknesses like coronary illness and type 2 diabetes and hypertension. Truth be told, when you eat the average American eating routine that is brimming with creature items and handled nourishments, your cells become excited regardless of whether you don't understand it. This cell irritation makes the body age quicker, as per a few investigations. The most ideal approach to keep away from this kind of unfortunate aggravation and diminish the danger of infection is by eating a sound, spotless, entire nourishments, plant-based eating regimen. Studies demonstrate that leafy foods high in cell reinforcements, including papaya, help lessen this irritation.

You needn't bother with a great deal of leafy foods to have an effect on your wellbeing. In one investigation, a preliminary gathering of nonsmoking men burned-through 2 servings of foods grown from the ground for about a month, expanding their normal admission up 5 servings and afterward to 8 servings per day. Results found that a moderate admission of vegetables and organic products may decrease irritation as adequately as eating more leafy foods. So you can add 2 every day and get the advantages your body needs. In any case, the individuals who ate more enrolled more elevated levels of solid carotenoid and other disease battling compounds and were significantly better, yet on the off chance that the objective is to decrease aggravation, 2 servings daily takes care of business.

4. Papaya as Part of a High-Fiber Diet, Can Help You Lose Weight

Tropical natural product will in general be lower in fiber than good decisions like an apple, yet, papaya conveys all the pleasantness and fiber that you require when you need a sweet tidbit yet you are attempting to avoid added sugar. One little papaya contains 3 grams of fiber, making it an ideal expansion to a smoothie or acai bowl, and a simple evening nibble.

High-fiber nourishments are connected to weight reduction since they top you off and cause your body to consume calories gradually. The solvent fiber in papaya hinders the absorption pace of different supplements (like starches that you eat) and forestalls sharp spikes in glucose, thusly you feel full faster and stay full more, which makes it simpler to get in shape, as indicated by research. What's more, in light of the fact that your body isn't quickly processing food, when you eat high-fiber food sources like papaya, you will not experience a sugar crash or feel hungry not long after eating.

5. Papaya May Protect Against Damage and Help You Achieve Youthful-Looking Skin

For more youthful looking skin that doesn't show harm from the sun or other ecological components, eating papaya can go back in time, since its significant degrees of nutrient C and lycopene go about as strong cell reinforcements that have been demonstrated to help lessen indications of maturing. These two amazing mixtures are known for their enemy of maturing properties.

Nutrient C animates collagen development and collagen is the hidden design of your skin. It likewise shields your skin cells against harm from UV light, as indicated by an investigation.

Lycopene is known to lessen wrinkles by making skin smoother. In an examination, post-menopausal ladies devoured an enhancement of lycopene and nutrient C, and following 14 weeks they found that their wrinkles had become smoother and their appearances more youthful looking. This might be one explanation that numerous regular skincare products incorporate papaya extract for its smooth, clear skin properties.

The body's maturing cycle begins at 30 years old, sooner than you may have anticipated. One approach to moderate the effect of maturing on your skin and body is to eat an eating routine plentiful in products of the soil add high fiber, nutrient pressed food sources like papaya to your plate

CHAPTER THREE

10 THINGS YOU CAN DO TO LOOSE WEIGHT SUCCESSFULLY

01. Instructions to follow to add weight

While restrictive dinner designs and centered energy wellbeing plans are a segment of the standard techniques for killing your headstrong fats and losing a couple of inches, there are certain lifestyle changes that can in like manner empower your weight decrease desires. Shedding pounds can be a task, yet not with the exception of in the event that you make little adjusts to your eating routine plans and standard timetables. Taking everything into account, here are 10 things you can do or change in your regular daily existence that can help you with shedding pounds sufficiently and gainfully.

02. Drink a great deal of water

Water is one of the crucial wellsprings of energy in our body. It improves your absorption just as collects your invulnerable structure. Beside that, it helps your weight decrease destinations by keeping you fulfilled for a more drawn out time span and helping you with avoiding unwanted carbs and fats.

03. Rest adequately

Various investigates have stated a connection between rest constraint and negative changes in assimilation, which can consistently provoke weight get. In light of everything, it is huge that you get sufficient trust the evidence speak for itself, on the

off chance that you're expecting to lose
some weight.

04. Add sound fats to your eating schedule

People who are expecting to lose some
weight much of the time detested fats. In
any case, in case you add supplement rich
unsaturated fats to your eating routine, it
can assemble the impression of finish in you
and keep you from insatiably devouring
food unfortunate fats later.

05. Abatement the proportion of oil in cooking

On the off chance that you're genuinely
expecting to lose a couple of inches, you
ought to oblige more unassuming
proportions of oil in your cooking. While a
couple of oils, like avocado or sunflower oil,

are more grounded than others and certain oils are affluent in sound fats, you should keep a psyche the substance of oil you use in your cooking.

06. Eat more fiber

By growing the substance of fiber in your eating schedule, you're improving your stomach related prosperity, yet moreover reducing the proportion of calorie confirmation, as fiber causes you stay full for a more expanded time span. Common items, green vegetables, nuts, whole grains, beans, and vegetables are some amazing wellsprings of fiber.

07. Addition your protein confirmation

Protein is a huge wellspring of energy in your body. Adding protein to your morning feast diet or some other supper can help manufacture muscles, yet moreover makes you full for the entire day, diminishing the amount of calorie utilization.

08. Consume more vegetables

In case you wish to get fit as a fiddle, you should add more vegetables to your eating schedule. Green vegetables are unprecedented wellsprings of strong enhancements and supplements. Other than coordinating your glucose levels, it moreover gives you the impression of consummation and empowers you cut down on undesirable sustenances.

Solidifying it with different dinners and diets will simply help you with getting fit as a fiddle enough.

09. Do whatever it takes not to ravenously burn-through food

Until and with the exception of in case you're glutting on the sound goodies, you should avoid it whatever amount of you can. Unwanted chomps may have all the earmarks of being tempting yet the thing extends the level of body fats in your body. Consequently, quit snacking up on things that will simply incite mourn later on.

10. Change to omega-3-rich food sources

Omega-3-rich food sources, for instance, oily fishes help you achive weight decrease destinations. Investigation has found that omega-3-rich sustenances can help cut back stomach fat and moreover increase metabolic rate.

CHAPTER FOUR

GOLO DIET

What is the GOLO diet? Would it have the option to help you with shedding pounds?

There are many weight decrease checks calories you can peruse while meaning to get more fit. GOLO diet was one of the top glanced through weight control plans of 2016 and continues making buzz. Here is all you need to consider the GOLO diet if you are needing to endeavor it.

What is the GOLO diet?

Rather than limiting carbs, fats or some other enhancement, the GOLO diet bases on changing the synthetics. The perspective behind the eating routine is that hormonal disparity can trigger anxiety, stress which can provoke vulnerable rest, longing for and exhaustion. This subsequently can provoke unfortunate weight secure.

The producers of the GOLO diet acknowledge that diet and exercise alone can't have suffering weight decrease impacts. To improve these eating routine affinities, the producers of the eating routine settled on a case they decision Release, which is a huge piece of the eating routine.

The GOLO diet supplement

Conveyance, the improvement contains critical plant eliminates and the key minerals that have been exhibited to assist manage the physical and mental piece of weight. It improves glucose levels, insulin rule, balance synthetics and extends hunger and control desires.

The improvement is taken with dinners and the part is lesser in case you simply need to lose essentially 5 to 10 kilos.

As shown by the National Medicine Comprehension Database, a couple of trimmings in the conveyance may trigger squeamishness or upset digestion.

What sustenances would you have the option to eat when on a GOLO diet?

One of the huge food parts of the GOLO diet is the GOLO Metabolic Fuel Matrix, which licenses you to make judgments from four fuel social affairs - protein, carbs, fats and vegetables.

Rehearsing can help you with getting centers, where you can consume extra snacks for the span of the day.

Here is an overview of sustenances you are asked to eat

Protein: Eggs, meat, poultry, fish, nuts and dairy things.

Carbs: Berries, natural items, sweet potatoes, white potatoes, beans and whole grains.

Vegetables: Broccoli, spinach, kale, sprouts, cauliflower, celery, cucumber, zucchini

Fats: Olive oil, coconut oil, chia seeds, hemp seeds, flax seeds.

GOLO plate of blended greens dressings

You should eat three dinners every day and are assigned 1-2 standard servings of each fuel pack per feast.

Will the eating routine help you with getting more slender?

The eating routine backings eating whole sustenances and extending exercise that can help overall weight decrease. The examinations done about the eating routine are by the genuine association and henceforth have a high risk of tendency.

Sustenances to avoid the eating routine cripple arranged and refined sustenances and spotlights on eating whole food sources taking everything into account.

Here are a couple of food sources you should avoid in GOLO diet

Arranged food sources: Potato chips, treats, wafers and warmed items

Red meat: Fatty cuts, cheeseburger, sheep, pork

Sugar-improved rewards: Soda, sports drinks, improved teas, supplement waters and crushes

Grains: Bread, grain, rice, oats, pasta, millet

Dairy things: Cheese, milk, yogurt, margarine, frozen yogurt

Fake sugars: Saccharin, aspartame and sucralose.

CHAPTER FIVE

A Game Changer

Drug Brings Weight Loss in Patients With Obesity.

Ana maria shed 40 pounds while participating in a clinical fundamental of the medicine semaglutide. "It should be the meds," she said. Exactly when the starter completed, her weight started to slither up. Ana Maria shed 40 pounds while looking into a clinical fundamental of the drug semaglutide. "It should be the drugs," she said. Right when the primer completed, her weight started to slither up.

Suddenly, a prescription has been demonstrated so incredible against robustness that patients may stay away from a significant parcel of its most perceptibly terrible outcomes, including diabetes.

The prescription, semaglutide, made by Novo Nordisk, as of now is promoted as a treatment for Type 2 diabetes. In a clinical primer disseminated in the New England Journal of Medicine, researchers at Northwestern University in Chicago attempted semaglutide at significantly higher segment as an adversary of weight solution.

Right around 2,000 individuals, at 129 concentrations in 16 countries, imbued themselves step by step with semaglutide or a phony treatment for 68 weeks. Overall, differentiated and 2.4 percent among those tolerating the phony treatment.

In abundance of 33% of the individuals getting the drug lost in overabundance of 20% of their weight. Signs of diabetes and pre-diabetes improved in various patients.

Those results far outperform the proportion of weight decrease saw in clinical fundamentals of other heftiness drugs, experts said. The drug is a "particular benefit," said Dr. Robert F. Kushner, a heaviness researcher at Northwestern University Feinberg School of Medicine, who drove the assessment. "This is the start of another time of fruitful drugs for weight."

Dr. Clifford Rosen of Maine Medical Center Research Institute, who was not related with the fundamental, said, "I think it has an enormous potential for weight decrease." Gastrointestinal results among the individuals were "really irrelevant — not the slightest bit like with weight decrease tranquilizes previously," added Dr. Rosen, an editor at the New England Journal of Medicine and a co-author of an article going with the assessment.

For a serious long time, analysts have searched for ways to deal with help creating amounts of people fighting with weight. Five at present available foe of heftiness drugs have results that limit their use. By and large, and can be taken remarkably for a short period of time. After it is ended, even that proportion of weight is recovered.

All things considered, noted Dr. Louis Aronne, a beefiness expert at Weill Cornell Medicine in New York who urges Novo Nordisk and studies semaglutide.

However, operation is a prominent course of action that forever changes the stomach related system. Only 1% of the people who qualify continue with the procedure. In light of everything, most enormous people endeavor a lot more than one eating routine with baffling results.

The semaglutide study avows what specialists certainly know, Dr. Kushner said: Willpower isn't adequate. In the new starter, individuals who got the phony treatment and diet and exercise exhorting couldn't see any basic difference in their weight.

Generally, back up plans have wouldn't pay for the weight decrease drugs accessible. Semaglutide is most likely going to be exorbitant. The lower parcel used to treat diabetes passes on an ordinary retail cost of nearly $1,000 consistently. (Back up plans ordinarily pay for diabetes drugs, Dr. Kushner noted.)

Dr. Caroline Apovian, co-top of the Center for Weight Management and Wellness at Brigham and Women's Hospital and a person from Novo Nordisk's notice board, said the sufficiency of semaglutide was "astounding" and that the primer results may lead wellbeing net suppliers to cover it.

Semaglutide is a produced variation of a typically happening substance that circles back to longing for networks in the psyche and in the gut, causing vibes of satiety. A high-partition routine of the medicine has not been focused long enough to know whether it has real long stretch results.

Moreover, it is typical that patients would have to take it for a lifetime to hold the weight decrease back from returning.

Ana Maria, who lives in Chicago, experienced years endeavoring to get fit as a fiddle with diets and drugs, anyway without quite a bit of any outcome. By then Ms. Ana joined the semaglutide fundamental and shed 40 pounds, around 15% of her weight.

Ms.Ana didn't know as yet whether she was getting the drug or the phony treatment. Regardless of the way that she was endeavoring to eat well and exercise, her weight "was dropping unreasonably brisk," she said. "It should be the drugs."

She experienced no outcomes, she said. Regardless, when the fundamental

completed and she not, now got the
medicine, the weight started returning. "I
was so melancholy," she said. She is on
edge to keep taking the drug once it's open

www.ingramcontent.com/pod-product-compliance
Lightning Source LLC
Chambersburg PA
CBHW060917130726
48001CB00006B/2280